MW01230425

Alkaline Side Dish Cookbook

50 Tasty and Clean Side Dish Recipes for your Alkaline Diet

Isaac Vinson

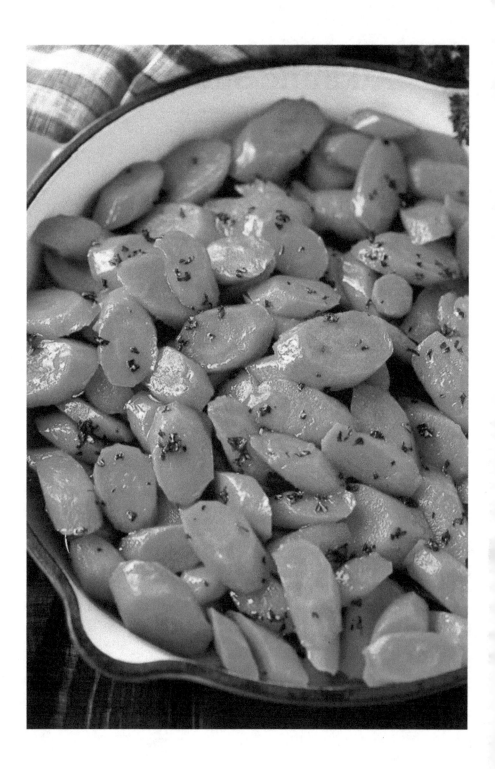

Table of Contents

Coffee-Steamed Carrots

Preparation Time: 10 minutes
Cooking Time: 3 minutes
Servings: 4

Ingredients :

• 1 cup brewed coffee

• 1 teaspoon light brown sugar

• ½ teaspoon kosher salt

• Freshly ground black pepper

• 1-pound baby carrots

• Chopped fresh parsley

• 1 teaspoon grated lemon zest

Directions:

1. Pour the coffee into the electric pressure cooker. Stir in the brown sugar, salt, and pepper. Add the carrots.

2. Close the pressure cooker. Set to sealing.

3. Cook on high pressure for minutes.

4. Once complete, click Cancel and quick release the pressure.

5. Once the pin drops, open and remove the lid.

6. Using a slotted spoon, portion carrots to a serving bowl. Topped with the parsley and lemon zest, and serve.

Nutrition:

51 Calories

12g Carbohydrates

4g Fiber

Rosemary Potatoes

Preparation Time: 5 minutes

Cooking Time: 25 minutes

Servings: 2

Ingredients :

• 1lb red potatoes

• 1 cup vegetable stock

• 2tbsp olive oil

• 2tbsp rosemary sprigs

Directions:

1. Situate potatoes in the steamer basket and add the stock into the Instant Pot.

2. Steam the potatoes in your Instant Pot for 15 minutes.

3. Depressurize and pour away the remaining stock.

4. Set to sauté and add the oil, rosemary, and potatoes.

5. Cook until brown.

Nutrition:

195 Calories

31g Carbohydrates

1g Fat

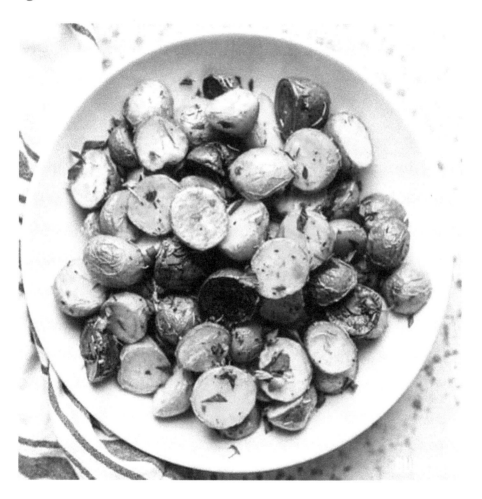

Corn on the Cob

Preparation Time: 10 minutes

Cooking Time: 5 minutes

Servings: 12

Ingredients :

• 6 ears corn

Directions:

1. Take off husks and silk from the corn. Cut or break each ear in half.

2. Pour 1 cup of water into the bottom of the electric pressure cooker. Insert a wire rack or trivet.

3. Place the corn upright on the rack, cut-side down. Seal lid of the pressure cooker.

4. Cook on high pressure for 5 minutes.

5. When its complete, select Cancel and quick release the pressure.

6. When pin drops, unlock and take off lid.

7. Pull out the corn from the pot. Season as desired and serve immediately.

Nutrition:

62 Calories

14g Carbohydrates

1g Fiber

Chili Lime Salmon

Preparation Time: 6 minutes
Cooking Time: 10 minutes
Servings: 2

Ingredients :

For Sauce:

- 1 jalapeno pepper

- 1 tablespoon chopped parsley

- 1 teaspoon minced garlic

- 1/2 teaspoon cumin

- 1/2 teaspoon paprika

- 1/2 teaspoon lime zest

- 1 tablespoon honey

- 1 tablespoon lime juice

- 1 tablespoon olive oil

- 1 tablespoon water

For Fish:

- 2 salmon fillets, each about 5 ounces

- 1 cup water

- 1/2 teaspoon salt

- 1/8 teaspoon ground black pepper

Directions:

1. Prepare salmon and for this, season salmon with salt and black pepper until evenly coated.

2. Plugin instant pot, insert the inner pot, pour in water, then place steamer basket and place seasoned salmon on it.

3. Seal instant pot with its lid, press the 'steam' button, then press the 'timer' to set the cooking time to 5 minutes and cook on high pressure, for 5 minutes.

4. Transfer all the Ingredients for the sauce in a bowl, whisk until combined and set aside until required.

5. When the timer beeps, press 'cancel' button and do quick pressure release until pressure nob drops down.

6. Open the instant pot, then transfer salmon to a serving plate and drizzle generously with prepared sauce.

7. Serve straight away.

Nutrition:

305 Calories

29g Carbohydrates

6g Fiber

Mashed Pumpkin

Preparation Time: 9 minutes

Cooking Time: 15 minutes

Servings: 2

Ingredients :

- 2 cups chopped pumpkin

- 0.5 cup water

- 2tbsp powdered sugar-free sweetener of choice

- 1tbsp cinnamon

Directions:

1. Place the pumpkin and water in your Instant Pot.

2. Seal and cook on Stew 15 minutes.

3. Remove and mash with the sweetener and cinnamon.

Nutrition:

12 Calories

3g Carbohydrates

1g Sugar

Parmesan-Topped Acorn Squash

Preparation Time: 8 minutes

Cooking Time: 20 minutes

Servings: 4

Ingredients :

• 1 acorn squash (about 1 pound)

• 1 tablespoon extra-virgin olive oil

• 1 teaspoon dried sage leaves, crumbled

• ¼ teaspoon freshly grated nutmeg

• 1/8 teaspoon kosher salt

• 1/8 teaspoon freshly ground black pepper

• 2 tablespoons freshly grated Parmesan cheese

Directions:

1. Chop acorn squash in half lengthwise and remove the seeds. Cut each half in half for a total of 4 wedges. Snap off the stem if it's easy to do.

2. In a small bowl, combine the olive oil, sage, nutmeg, salt, and pepper. Brush the cut sides of the squash with the olive oil mixture.

3. Fill 1 cup of water into the electric pressure cooker and insert a wire rack or trivet.

4. Place the squash on the trivet in a single layer, skin-side down.

5. Set the lid of the pressure cooker on sealing.

6. Cook on high pressure for 20 minutes.

7. Once done, press Cancel and quick release the pressure.

8. Once the pin drops, open it.

9. Carefully remove the squash from the pot, sprinkle with the Parmesan, and serve.

Nutrition:

85 Calories

12g Carbohydrates

2g Fiber

Quinoa Tabbouleh

Preparation Time: 8 minutes

Cooking Time: 16 minutes

Servings: 6

Ingredients :

• 1 cup quinoa, rinsed

• 1 large English cucumber

• 2 scallions, sliced

• 2 cups cherry tomatoes, halved

• **Servings:** cup chopped parsley

• 1/2 cup chopped mint

• ½ teaspoon minced garlic

• 1/2 teaspoon salt

• ½ teaspoon ground black pepper

• 2 tablespoon lemon juice

• 1/2 cup olive oil

Directions:

1. Plugin instant pot, insert the inner pot, add quinoa, then pour in water and stir until mixed.

2. Close instant pot with its lid and turn the pressure knob to seal the pot.

3. Select 'manual' button, then set the 'timer' to 1 minute and cook in high pressure, it may take 7 minutes.

4. Once the timer stops, select 'cancel' button and do natural pressure release for 10 minutes and then do quick pressure release until pressure nob drops down.

5. Open the instant pot, fluff quinoa with a fork, then spoon it on a rimmed baking sheet, spread quinoa evenly and let cool.

6. Meanwhile, place lime juice in a small bowl, add garlic and stir until just mixed.

7. Then add salt, black pepper, and olive oil and whisk until combined.

8. Transfer cooled quinoa to a large bowl, add remaining Ingredients, then drizzle generously with the prepared lime juice mixture and toss until evenly coated.

9. Taste quinoa to adjust seasoning and then serve.

Nutrition:

283 Calories

30.6g Carbohydrates

3. 4g Fiber

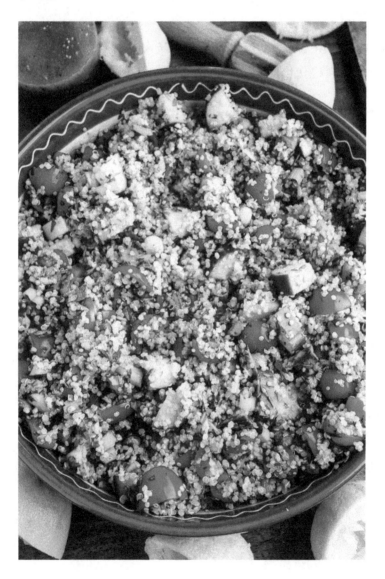

Wild Rice Salad with Cranberries and Almonds

Preparation Time: 6 minutes

Cooking Time: 25 minutes

Servings: 18

Ingredients :

For the rice

• 2 cups wild rice blend, rinsed

• 1 teaspoon kosher salt

• 2½ cups Vegetable Broth

For the dressing

• ¼ cup extra-virgin olive oil

• ¼ cup white wine vinegar

• 1½ teaspoons grated orange zest

• Juice of 1 medium orange (about ¼ cup)

• 1 teaspoon honey or pure maple syrup

For the salad

• ¾ cup unsweetened dried cranberries

- ½ cup sliced almonds, toasted

- Freshly ground black pepper

Directions:

1. To make the rice

2. In the electric pressure cooker, combine the rice, salt, and broth.

3. Close and lock the lid. Set the valve to sealing.

4. Cook on high pressure for 25 minutes.

5. When the cooking is complete, hit Cancel and allow the pressure to release naturally for 1minutes, then quick release any remaining pressure.

6. Once the pin drops, unlock and remove the lid.

7. Let the rice cool briefly, then fluff it with a fork.

8. To make the dressing

9. While the rice cooks, make the dressing: In a small jar with a screw-top lid, combine the olive oil, vinegar, zest, juice, and honey. (If you don't have a jar, whisk the Ingredients together in a small bowl.) Shake to combine.

10. To make the salad

11. Mix rice, cranberries, and almonds.

12. Add the dressing and season with pepper.

13. Serve warm or refrigerate.

Nutrition

126 Calories

18g Carbohydrates

2g Fiber

Low Fat Roasties

Preparation Time: 8 minutes

Cooking Time: 25 minutes

Servings: 2

Ingredients :

• 1lb roasting potatoes

• 1 garlic clove

• 1 cup vegetable stock

• 2tbsp olive oil

Directions:

1. Position potatoes in the steamer basket and add the stock into the Instant Pot.

2. Steam the potatoes in your Instant Pot for 15 minutes.

3. Depressurize and pour away the remaining stock.

4. Set to sauté and add the oil, garlic, and potatoes. Cook until brown.

Nutrition:

201 Calories

3g Carbohydrates

6g Fat

Roasted Parsnips

Preparation Time: 9 minutes

Cooking Time: 25 minutes

Servings: 2

Ingredients :

• 1lb parsnips

• 1 cup vegetable stock

• 2tbsp herbs

• 2tbsp olive oil

Directions:

1. Put the parsnips in the steamer basket and add the stock into the Instant Pot.

2. Steam the parsnips in your Instant Pot for 15 minutes.

3. Depressurize and pour away the remaining stock.

4. Set to sauté and add the oil, herbs and parsnips.

5. Cook until golden and crisp.

Nutrition:

130 Calories

14g Carbohydrates

4g Protein

Lower Carb Hummus

Preparation Time: 9 minutes

Cooking Time: 60 minutes

Servings: 2

Ingredients :

• 0.5 cup dry chickpeas

• 1 cup vegetable stock

• 1 cup pumpkin puree

• 2tbsp smoked paprika

• salt and pepper to taste

Directions:

1. Soak the chickpeas overnight.

2. Place the chickpeas and stock in the Instant Pot.

3. Cook on Beans 60 minutes.

4. Depressurize naturally.

5. Blend the chickpeas with the remaining Ingredients.

Nutrition:

135 Calories

18g Carbohydrates

3g Fat

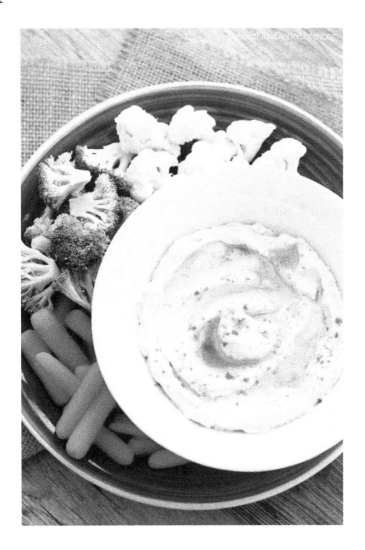

Sweet and Sour Red Cabbage

Preparation Time: 7 minutes
Cooking Time: 10 minutes
Servings: 8

Ingredients :

• 2 cups Spiced Pear Applesauce

• 1 small onion, chopped

• ½ cup apple cider vinegar

• ½ teaspoon kosher salt

• 1 head red cabbage

Directions:

1. In the electric pressure cooker, combine the applesauce, onion, vinegar, salt, and cup of water. Stir in the cabbage.

2. Seal lid of the pressure cooker.

3. Cook on high pressure for 10 minutes.

4. When the cooking is complete, hit Cancel and quick release the pressure.

5. Once the pin drops, unlock and remove the lid.

6. Spoon into a bowl or platter and serve.

Nutrition:

91 Calories

18g Carbohydrates

4g Fiber

Pinto Beans

Preparation Time: 6 minutes
Cooking Time: 55 minutes
Servings: 10

Ingredients :

• 2 cups pinto beans, dried

• 1 medium white onion

• 1 ½ teaspoon minced garlic

• ¾ teaspoon salt

• 1/4 teaspoon ground black pepper

• 1 teaspoon red chili powder

• 1/4 teaspoon cumin

• 1 tablespoon olive oil

• 1 teaspoon chopped cilantro

• 5 ½ cup vegetable stock

Directions:

1. Plugin instant pot, insert the inner pot, press sauté/simmer button, add oil and when hot, add onion and garlic and cook for 3 minutes or until onions begin to soften.

2. Add remaining Ingredients, stir well, then press the cancel button, shut the instant pot with its lid and seal the pot.

3. Click 'manual' button, then press the 'timer' to set the cooking time to 45 minutes and cook at high pressure.

4. Once done, click 'cancel' button and do natural pressure release for 10 minutes until pressure nob drops down.

5. Open the instant pot, spoon beans into plates and serve.

Nutrition:

107 Calories

11. 7g Carbohydrates

4g Fiber

Parmesan Cauliflower Mash

Preparation Time: 19 minutes

Cooking Time: 5 minutes

Servings: 4

Ingredients :

• 1 head cauliflower

• ½ teaspoon kosher salt

• ½ teaspoon garlic pepper

• 2 tablespoons plain Greek yogurt

• ¾ cup freshly grated Parmesan cheese

• 1 tablespoon unsalted butter or ghee (optional)

• Chopped fresh chives

Directions:

1. Pour cup of water into the electric pressure cooker and insert a steamer basket or wire rack.

2. Place the cauliflower in the basket.

3. Cover lid of the pressure cooker to seal.

4. Cook on high pressure for 5 minutes.

5. Once complete, hit Cancel and quick release the pressure.

6. When the pin drops, remove the lid.

7. Remove the cauliflower from the pot and pour out the water. Return the cauliflower to the pot and add the salt, garlic pepper, yogurt, and cheese. Use an immersion blender to purée or mash the cauliflower in the pot.

8. Spoon into a serving bowl, and garnish with butter (if using) and chives.

Nutrition:

141 Calories

12g Carbohydrates

4g Fiber

Steamed Asparagus

Preparation Time: 3 minutes

Cooking Time: 2 minutes

Servings: 4

Ingredients :

• 1 lb. fresh asparagus, rinsed and tough ends trimmed

• 1 cup water

Directions:

1. Place the asparagus into a wire steamer rack, and set it inside your Instant Pot.

2. Add water to the pot. Close and seal the lid, turning the steam release valve to the "Sealing" position.

3. Select the "Steam" function to cook on high pressure for 2 minutes.

4. Once done, do a quick pressure release of the steam.

5. Lift the wire steamer basket out of the pot and place the asparagus onto a serving plate.

6. Season as desired and serve.

Nutrition:

22 Calories

4g Carbohydrates

2g Protein

Squash Medley

Preparation Time: 10 minutes
Cooking Time: 20 minutes.

Servings: 2

Ingredients :

• 2 lbs. mixed squash

• ½ cup mixed veg

• 1 cup vegetable stock

• 2 tbsps. olive oil

• 2 tbsps. mixed herbs

Direction:

1. Put the squash in the steamer basket and add the stock into the Instant Pot.

2. Steam the squash in your Instant Pot for 10 minutes.

3. Depressurize and pour away the remaining stock.

4. Set to sauté and add the oil and remaining Ingredients.

5. Cook until a light crust form.

Nutrition:

100 Calories

10g Carbohydrates

6g Fat

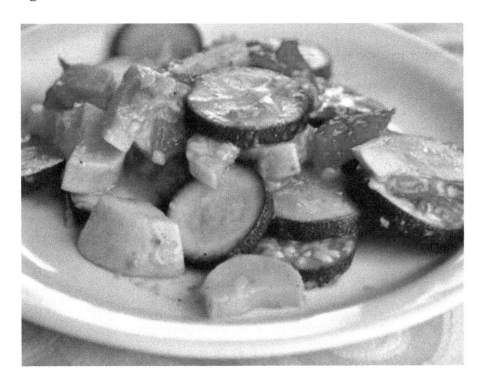

Eggplant Curry

Preparation Time: 15 minutes

Cooking Time: 20 minutes

Servings: 2

Ingredients :
- 3 cups chopped eggplant

- 1 thinly sliced onion

- 1 cup coconut milk

- 3 tbsps. curry paste

- 1 tbsp. oil or ghee

Directions:

1. Select Instant Pot to sauté and put the onion, oil, and curry paste.

2. Once the onion is soft, stir in remaining Ingredients and seal.

3. Cook on Stew for 20 minutes. Release the pressure naturally.

Nutrition:

350 Calories

15g Carbohydrates

25g Fat

Lentil and Eggplant Stew

Preparation Time: 15 minutes
Cooking Time: 35 minutes
Servings: 2

Ingredients :

• 1 lb. eggplant

• 1 lb. dry lentils

• 1 cup chopped vegetables

• 1 cup low sodium vegetable broth

Directions:

1. Incorporate all the Ingredients in your Instant Pot, cook on Stew for 35 minutes.

2. Release the pressure naturally and serve.

Nutrition:

310 Calories

22g Carbohydrates

10g Fat

Lentil and Chickpea Curry

Preparation Time: 15 minutes

Cooking Time: 20 minutes

Servings: 2

Ingredients :

- 2 cups dry lentils and chickpeas

- 1 thinly sliced onion

- 1 cup chopped tomato

- 3 tbsps. curry paste

- 1 tbsp. oil or ghee

Directions:

1. Press Instant Pot to sauté and mix onion, oil, and curry paste.

2. Once the onion is cooked, stir the remaining Ingredients and seal.

3. Cook on Stew for 20 minutes.

4. Release the pressure naturally and serve.

Nutrition:

360 Calories

26g Carbohydrates

19g Fat

Split Pea Stew

Preparation Time: 5 minutes

Cooking Time: 35 minutes

Servings: 2

Ingredients :

• 1 cup dry split peas

• 1 lb. chopped vegetables

• 1 cup mushroom soup

• 2 tbsps. old bay seasoning

Directions:

1. Incorporate all the Ingredients in Instant Pot, cook for 33 minutes.

2. Release the pressure naturally.

Nutrition:

300 Calories

7g Carbohydrates

2g Fat

Fried Tofu Hotpot

Preparation Time: 15 minutes
Cooking Time: 15 minutes
Servings: 2

Ingredients :

• ½ lb. fried tofu

• 1 lb. chopped Chinese vegetable mix

• 1 cup low sodium vegetable broth

• 2 tbsps. 5 spice seasoning

• 1 tbsp. smoked paprika

Direction:

1. Combine all the Ingredients in your Instant Pot, set on Stew for 15 minutes.

2. Release the pressure naturally and serve.

Nutrition:

320 Calories

11g Carbohydrates

23g Fat

Chili Sin Carne

Preparation Time: 15 minutes

Cooking Time: 35 minutes

Servings: 2

Ingredients :

• 3 cups mixed cooked beans

• 2 cups chopped tomatoes

• 1 tbsp. yeast extract

• 2 squares very dark chocolate

• 1 tbsp. red chili flakes

Directions:

1. Combine all the Ingredients in your Instant Pot, cook for 35 minutes.

2. Release the pressure naturally and serve.

Nutrition:

240 Calories

20g Carbohydrates

3g Fat

Brussels Sprouts

Preparation Time: 5 minutes

Cooking Time: 3 minutes

Servings: 5

Ingredients :

• 1 tsp. extra-virgin olive oil

• 1 lb. halved Brussels sprouts

• 3 tbsps. apple cider vinegar

• 3 tbsps. gluten-free tamari soy sauce

• 3 tbsps. chopped sun-dried tomatoes

Directions:

1. Select the "Sauté" function on your Instant Pot, add oil and allow the pot to get hot.

2. Cancel the "Sauté" function and add the Brussels sprouts.

3. Stir well and allow the sprouts to cook in the residual heat for 2-3 minutes.

4. Add the tamari soy sauce and vinegar, and then stir.

5. Cover the Instant Pot, sealing the pressure valve by pointing it to "Sealing."

6. Select the "Manual, High Pressure" setting and cook for 3 minutes.

7. Once the cook cycle is done, do a quick pressure release, and then stir in the chopped sun-dried tomatoes.

8. Serve immediately.

Nutrition:

62 Calories

10g Carbohydrates

1g Fat

Garlic and Herb Carrots

Preparation Time: 2 minutes

Cooking Time: 18 minutes

Servings: 3

Ingredients :

• 2 tbsps. butter

• 1 lb. baby carrots

• 1 cup water

• 1 tsp. fresh thyme or oregano

• 1 tsp. minced garlic

• Black pepper

• Coarse sea salt

Directions:

1. Fill water to the inner pot of the Instant Pot, and then put in a steamer basket.

2. Layer the carrots into the steamer basket.

3. Close and seal the lid, with the pressure vent in the "Sealing" position.

4. Select the "Steam" setting and cook for 2 minutes on high pressure.

5. Quick release the pressure and then carefully remove the steamer basket with the steamed carrots, discarding the water.

6. Add butter to the inner pot of the Instant Pot and allow it to melt on the "Sauté" function.

7. Add garlic and sauté for 30 seconds, and then add the carrots. Mix well.

8. Stir in the fresh herbs, and cook for 2-3 minutes.

9. Season with salt and black pepper, and the transfer to a serving bowl.

10. Serve warm and enjoy!

Nutrition:

122 Calories

12g Carbohydrates

7g Fat

Cilantro Lime Drumsticks

Preparation Time: 5 minutes
Cooking Time: 15 minutes
Servings: 6

Ingredients :

• 1 tbsp. olive oil

• 6 chicken drumsticks

• 4 minced garlic cloves

• ½ cup low-sodium chicken broth

• 1 tsp. cayenne pepper

• 1 tsp. crushed red peppers

• 1 tsp. fine sea salt

• Juice of 1 lime

To Serve:

• 2 tbsp. chopped cilantro

• Extra lime zest

Directions:

1. Pour olive oil to the Instant Pot and set it on the "Sauté" function.

2. Once the oil is hot adding the chicken drumsticks, and season them well.

3. Using tongs, stir the drumsticks and brown the drumsticks for 2 minutes per side.

4. Add the lime juice, fresh cilantro, and chicken broth to the pot.

5. Lock and seal the lid, turning the pressure valve to "Sealing."

6. Cook the drumsticks on the "Manual, High Pressure" setting for 9 minutes.

7. Once done let the pressure release naturally.

8. Carefully transfer the drumsticks to an aluminum-foiled baking sheet and broil them in the oven for 3-5 minutes until golden brown.

9. Serve warm, garnished with more cilantro and lime zest.

Nutrition:

480 Calories

3.3g Carbohydrates

29g Fat

Eggplant Spread

Preparation Time: 5 minutes
Cooking Time: 18 minutes
Servings: 5

Ingredients :

• 4 tbsps. extra-virgin olive oil

• 2 lbs. eggplant

• 4 skin-on garlic cloves

• ½ cup water

• ¼ cup pitted black olives

• 3 sprigs fresh thyme

• Juice of 1 lemon

• 1 tbsp. tahini

• 1 tsp. sea salt

• Fresh extra-virgin olive oil

Directions:

1. Peel the eggplant in alternating stripes, leaving some areas with skin and some with no skin.

2. Slice into big chunks and layer at the bottom of your Instant Pot.

3. Add olive oil to the pot, and on the "Sauté" function, fry and caramelize the eggplant on one side, about 5 minutes.

4. Add in the garlic cloves with the skin on.

5. Flip over the eggplant and then add in the remaining uncooked eggplant chunks, salt, and water.

6. Close the lid, ensure the pressure release valve is set to "Sealing."

7. Cook for 5 minutes on the "Manual, High Pressure" setting.

8. Once done, carefully open the pot by quick releasing the pressure through the steam valve.

9. Discard most of the brown cooking liquid.

10. Remove the garlic cloves and peel them.

11. Add the lemon juice, tahini, cooked and fresh garlic cloves and pitted black olives to the pot.

12. Using a hand-held immersion blender, process all the Ingredients until smooth.

13. Pour out the spread into a serving dish and season with fresh thyme, whole black olives and some extra-virgin olive oil, prior to serving.

Nutrition:

155 Calories

16.8g Carbohydrates

11. 7g Fat

Carrot Hummus

Preparation Time: 15 minutes

Cooking Time: 10 minutes

Servings: 2

Ingredients :

- 1 chopped carrot

- 2 oz. cooked chickpeas

- 1 tsp. lemon juice

- 1 tsp. tahini

- 1 tsp. fresh parsley

Directions:

1. Place the carrot and chickpeas in your Instant Pot.

2. Add a cup of water, seal, cook for 10 minutes on Stew.

3. Depressurize naturally. Blend with the remaining Ingredients.

Nutrition:

58 Calories

8g Carbohydrates

2g Fat

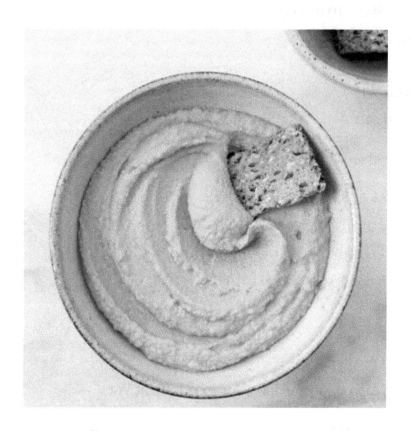

Vegetable Rice Pilaf

Preparation Time: 5 minutes
Cooking Time: 25 minutes
Servings: 6

Ingredients :
- 1 tablespoon olive oil

- ½ medium yellow onion, diced

- 1 cup uncooked long-grain brown rice

- 2 cloves minced garlic

- ½ teaspoon dried basil

- Salt and pepper

- 2 cups fat-free chicken broth

- 1 cup frozen mixed veggies

Directions:

1. Cook oil in a large skillet over medium heat.

2. Add the onion and sauté for 3 minutes until translucent.

3. Stir in the rice and cook until lightly toasted.

4. Add the garlic, basil, salt, and pepper then stir to combined.

5. Stir in the chicken broth then bring to a boil.

6. Decrease heat and simmer, covered, for 10 minutes.

7. Stir in the frozen veggies then cover and cook for another 10 minutes until heated through. Serve hot.

Nutrition:

90 Calories

12.6g Carbohydrates

2.2g Fiber

Curry Roasted Cauliflower Florets

Preparation Time: 5 minutes

Cooking Time: 25 minutes

Servings: 6

Ingredients :

• 8 cups cauliflower florets

• 2 tablespoons olive oil

• 1 teaspoon curry powder

• ½ teaspoon garlic powder

• Salt and pepper

Directions:

1. Prep the oven to 425°F and line a baking sheet with foil.

2. Toss the cauliflower with the olive oil and spread on the baking sheet.

3. Sprinkle with curry powder, garlic powder, salt, and pepper.

4. Roast for 25 minutes or until just tender. Serve hot.

Nutrition:

75 Calories

7.4g Carbohydrates

3.5g Fiber

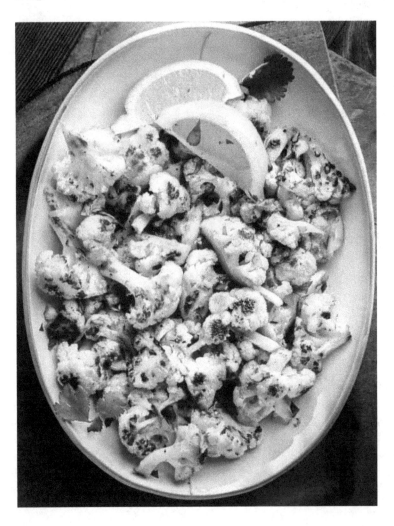

Mushroom Barley Risotto

Preparation Time: 5 minutes

Cooking Time: 25 minutes

Servings: 8

Ingredients :

• 4 cups fat-free beef broth

• 2 tablespoons olive oil

• 1 small onion, diced well

• 2 cloves minced garlic

• 8 ounces thinly sliced mushrooms

• ¼ tsp dried thyme

• Salt and pepper

• 1 cup pearled barley

• ½ cup dry white wine

Directions:

1. Heat the beef broth in a medium saucepan and keep it warm.

2. Heat the oil in a large, deep skillet over medium heat.

3. Add the onions and garlic and sauté for 2 minutes then stir in the mushrooms and thyme.

4. Season with salt and pepper and sauté for 2 minutes more.

5. Add the barley and sauté for 1 minute then pour in the wine.

6. Ladle about ½ cup of beef broth into the skillet and stir well to combine.

7. Cook until most of the broth has been absorbed then add another ladle.

8. Repeat until you have used all of the broth and the barley is cooked to al dente.

9. Season and serve hot.

Nutrition:

155 Calories

22.9g Carbohydrates

4.4g Fiber

Braised Summer Squash

Preparation Time: 10 minutes

Cooking Time: 20 minutes

Servings: 6

Ingredients :

• 3 tablespoons olive oil

• 3 cloves minced garlic

• ¼ teaspoon crushed red pepper flakes

• 1-pound summer squash, sliced

• 1-pound zucchini, sliced

• 1 teaspoon dried oregano

• Salt and pepper

Directions:

1. Cook oil in a large skillet over medium heat.

2. Add the garlic and crushed red pepper and cook for 2 minutes.

3. Add the summer squash and zucchini and cook for 15 minutes, stirring often, until just tender.

4. Stir in the oregano then season with salt and pepper to taste. serve hot.

Nutrition:

90 Calories

6.2g Carbohydrates

1.8g Fiber

Lemon Garlic Green Beans

Preparation Time: 5 minutes

Cooking Time: 10 minutes

Servings: 6

Ingredients :

• 1 1/2 pounds green beans, trimmed

• 2 tablespoons olive oil

• 1 tablespoon fresh lemon juice

• 2 cloves minced garlic

• Salt and pepper

Directions:

1. Fill a large bowl with ice water and set aside.

2. Bring a pot of salted water to boil then add the green beans.

3. Cook for 3 minutes then drain and immediately place in the ice water.

4. Cool the beans completely then drain them well.

5. Heat the oil in a large skillet over medium-high heat.

6. Add the green beans, tossing to coat, then add the lemon juice, garlic, salt, and pepper.

7. Sauté for 3 minutes until the beans are tender-crisp then serve hot.

Nutrition:

Calories 75,

Total Fat 4.8g,

Saturated Fat 0.7g,

Total Carbs 8.5g,

Net Carbs 4.6g,

Protein 2.1g,

Sugar 1.7g,

Fiber 3.9g,

Sodium 7mg

Brown Rice & Lentil Salad

Preparation Time: 10 minutes

Cooking Time: 10 minutes

Servings: 4

Ingredients :

- 1 cup water

- 1/2 cup instant brown rice

- 2 tablespoons olive oil

- 2 tablespoons red wine vinegar

- 1 tablespoon Dijon mustard

- 1 tablespoon minced onion

- 1/2 teaspoon paprika

- Salt and pepper

- 1 (15-ounce) can brown lentils, rinsed and drained

- 1 medium carrot, shredded

- 2 tablespoons fresh chopped parsley

Directions:

1. Stir together the water and instant brown rice in a medium saucepan.

2. Bring to a boil then simmer for 10 minutes, covered.

3. Remove from heat and set aside while you prepare the salad.

4. Whisk together the olive oil, vinegar, Dijon mustard, onion, paprika, salt, and pepper in a medium bowl.

5. Toss in the cooked rice, lentils, carrots, and parsley.

6. Adjust seasoning to taste then stir well and serve warm.

Nutrition:

Calories 145,

Total Fat 7.7g,

Saturated Fat 1g,

Total Carbs 13.1g,

Net Carbs 10.9g,

Protein 6g,

Sugar 1g,

Fiber 2.2g,

Mashed Butternut Squash

Preparation Time: 5 minutes

Cooking Time: 25 minutes

Servings: 6

Ingredients :

• 3 pounds whole butternut squash (about 2 medium)

• 2 tablespoons olive oil

• Salt and pepper

Directions:

1. Preheat the oven to 400F and line a baking sheet with parchment.

2. Cut the squash in half and remove the seeds.

3. Cut the squash into cubes and toss with oil then spread on the baking sheet.

4. Roast for 25 minutes until tender then place in a food processor.

5. Blend smooth then season with salt and pepper to taste.

Nutrition:

Calories 90,

Total Fat 4.8g,

Saturated Fat 0.7g,

Total Carbs 12.3g,

Net Carbs 10.2g,

Protein 1.1g,

Sugar 2.3g,

Fiber 2.1g,

Sodium 4mg

Cilantro Lime Quinoa

Preparation Time: 5 minutes
Cooking Time: 25 minutes
Servings: 6

Ingredients :

• 1 cup uncooked quinoa

• 1 tablespoon olive oil

• 1 medium yellow onion, diced

• 2 cloves minced garlic

• 1 (4-ounce) can diced green chiles, drained

• 1 1/2 cups fat-free chicken broth

• ¾ cup fresh chopped cilantro

• 1/2 cup sliced green onion

• 2 tablespoons lime juice

• Salt and pepper

Directions:

1. Rinse the quinoa thoroughly in cool water using a fine mesh sieve.

2. Heat the oil in a large saucepan over medium heat.

3. Add the onion and sauté for 2 minutes then stir in the chile and garlic.

4. Cook for 1 minute then stir in the quinoa and chicken broth.

5. Bring to a boil then reduce heat and simmer, covered, until the quinoa absorbs the liquid – about 20 to 25 minutes.

6. Remove from heat then stir in the cilantro, green onions, and lime juice.

7. Season with salt and pepper to taste and serve hot.

Nutrition:

Calories 150,

Total Fat 4.1g,

Saturated Fat 0.5g,

Total Carbs 22.5g,

Net Carbs 19.8g,

Protein 6g,

Sugar 1.7g,

Fiber 2.7g,

Sodium 179mg

Oven-Roasted Veggies

Preparation Time: 5 minutes

Cooking Time: 25 minutes

Servings: 6

Ingredients :

• 1 pound cauliflower florets

• 1/2 pound broccoli florets

• 1 large yellow onion, cut into chunks

• 1 large red pepper, cored and chopped

• 2 medium carrots, peeled and sliced

• 2 tablespoons olive oil

• 2 tablespoons apple cider vinegar

• Salt and pepper

Directions:

1. Preheat the oven to 425F and line a large rimmed baking sheet with parchment.

2. Spread the veggies on the baking sheet and drizzle with oil and vinegar.

3. Toss well and season with salt and pepper.

4. Spread the veggies in a single layer then roast for 20 to 25 minutes, stirring every 10 minutes, until tender.

5. Adjust seasoning to taste and serve hot.

Nutrition:

Calories 100,

Total Fat 5g,

Saturated Fat 0.7g,

Total Carbs 12.4g,

Net Carbs 8.2g,

Protein 3.2g,

Sugar 5.5g,

Fiber 4.2g,

Sodium 51mg

Parsley Tabbouleh

Preparation Time: 5 minutes
Cooking Time: 25 minutes
Servings: 6

Ingredients :

• 1 cup water

• 1/2 cup bulgur

• ¼ cup fresh lemon juice

• 2 tablespoons olive oil

• 2 cloves minced garlic

• Salt and pepper

• 2 cups fresh chopped parsley

• 2 medium tomatoes, died

• 1 small cucumber, diced

• ¼ cup fresh chopped mint

Directions:

1. Bring the water and bulgur to a boil in a small saucepan then remove from heat.

2. Cover and let stand until the water is fully absorbed, about 25 minutes.

3. Meanwhile, whisk together the lemon juice, olive oil, garlic, salt, and pepper in a medium bowl.

4. Toss in the cooked bulgur along with the parsley, tomatoes, cucumber, and mint.

5. Season with salt and pepper to taste and serve.

Nutrition:

Calories 110,

Total Fat 5.3g,

Saturated Fat 0.9g,

Total Carbs 14.4g,

Net Carbs 10.5g,

Protein 3g,

Sugar 2.4g,

Fiber 3.9g,

Garlic Sautéed Spinach

Preparation Time: 5 minutes

Cooking Time: 10 minutes

Servings: 4

Ingredients :

- 1 1/2 tablespoons olive oil

- 4 cloves minced garlic

- 6 cups fresh baby spinach

- Salt and pepper

Directions:

1. Heat the oil in a large skillet over medium-high heat.

2. Add the garlic and cook for 1 minute.

3. Stir in the spinach and season with salt and pepper.

4. Sauté for 1 to 2 minutes until just wilted. Serve hot.

Nutrition:

Calories 60,

Total Fat 5.5g,

Saturated Fat 0.8g,

Total Carbs 2.6g,

Net Carbs 1.5g,

Protein 1.5g,

Sugar 0.2g,

Fiber 1.1g,

Sodium 36mg

French Lentils

Preparation Time: 5 minutes
Cooking Time: 25 minutes
Servings: 10

Ingredients :
- 2 tablespoons olive oil

- 1 medium onion, diced

- 1 medium carrot, peeled and diced

- 2 cloves minced garlic

- 5 1/2 cups water

- 2 ¼ cups French lentils, rinsed and drained

- 1 teaspoon dried thyme

- 2 small bay leaves

- Salt and pepper

Directions:

1. Heat the oil in a large saucepan over medium heat.

2. Add the onions, carrot, and garlic and sauté for 3 minutes.

3. Stir in the water, lentils, thyme, and bay leaves – season with salt.

4. Bring to a boil then reduce to a simmer and cook until tender, about 20 minutes.

5. Drain any excess water and adjust seasoning to taste. Serve hot.

Nutrition:

Calories 185,

Total Fat 3.3g,

Saturated Fat 0.5g,

Total Carbs 27.9g,

Net Carbs 14.2g,

Protein 11.4g,

Sugar 1.7g,

Fiber 13.7g,

Sodium 11mg

Grain-Free Berry Cobbler

Preparation Time: 5 minutes
Cooking Time: 25 minutes
Servings: 10

Ingredients :

• 4 cups fresh mixed berries

• 1/2 cup ground flaxseed

• ¼ cup almond meal

• ¼ cup unsweetened shredded coconut

• 1/2 tablespoon baking powder

• 1 teaspoon ground cinnamon

• ¼ teaspoon salt

• Powdered stevia, to taste

• 6 tablespoons coconut oil

Directions:

1. Preheat the oven to 375F and lightly grease a 10-inch cast-iron skillet.

2. Spread the berries on the bottom of the skillet.

3. Whisk together the dry Ingredients in a mixing bowl.

4. Cut in the coconut oil using a fork to create a crumbled mixture.

5. Spread the crumble over the berries and bake for 25 minutes until hot and bubbling.

6. Cool the cobbler for 5 to 10 minutes before serving.

Nutrition:

Calories 215

Total Fat 16.8g,

Saturated Fat 10.4g,

Total Carbs 13.1g,

Net Carbs 6.7g,

Protein 3.7g,

Sugar 5.3g,

Fiber 6.4g,

Sodium 61mg

Creamy Avocado-Broccoli Soup

Preparation Time: 10 minutes

Cooking Time: 15 minutes

Servings: 1-2

Ingredients :

• 2-3 flowers broccoli

• 1 small avocado

• 1 yellow onion

• 1 green or red pepper

• 1 celery stalk

• 2 cups vegetable broth (yeast-free)

• Celtic Sea Salt to taste

Directions:

Warmth vegetable stock (don't bubble). Include hacked onion and broccoli, and warm for a few minutes. At that point put in blender, include the avocado, pepper and celery and Blend until the soup is smooth (include some more water whenever wanted). Flavor and serve warm. Delicious!!

Nutrition:

Calories: 60g

Carbohydrates: 11g

Fat: 2 g

Protein: 2g

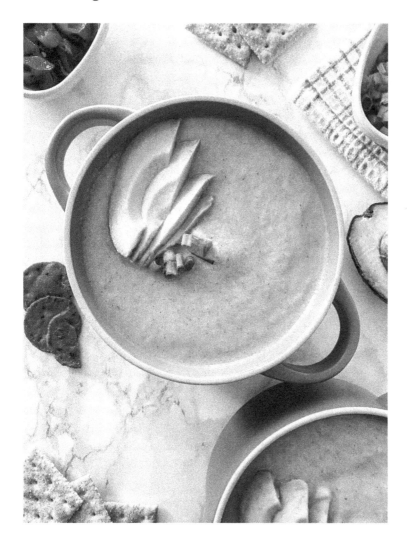

Fresh Garden Vegetable Soup

Preparation Time: 7 minutes
Cooking Time: 20 minutes
Servings: 1-2

Ingredients :

• 2 huge carrots

• 1 little zucchini

• 1 celery stem

• 1 cup of broccoli

• 3 stalks of asparagus

• 1 yellow onion

• 1 quart of (antacid) water

• 4-5 tsps. Of sans yeast vegetable stock

• 1 tsp. new basil

• 2 tsps. Ocean salt to taste

Directions:

1. Put water in pot, include the vegetable stock just as the onion and bring to bubble.

2. In the meantime, cleave the zucchini, the broccoli and the asparagus, and shred the carrots and the celery stem in a food processor.

3. When the water is bubbling, it would be ideal if you turn off the oven as we would prefer not to heat up the vegetables. Simply put them all in the high temp water and hold up until the vegetables arrive at wanted delicacy.

4. Permit to cool somewhat, at that point put all fixings into blender and blend until you get a thick, smooth consistency.

Nutrition:

Calories: 43

Carbohydrates: 7g

Fat: 1 g

Swiss Cauliflower-Emmenthal-Soup

Preparation Time: 10 minutes

Cooking Time: 15 minutes

Servings: 3-4

Ingredients :

• 2 cups cauliflower pieces

• 1 cup potatoes, cubed

• 2 cups vegetables stock (without yeast)

• 3 tbsp. Swiss Emmenthal cheddar, cubed

• 2 tbsp. new chives

• 1 tbsp. pumpkin seeds

• 1 touch of nutmeg and cayenne pepper

Directions:

1. Cook cauliflower and potato in vegetable stock until delicate and Blend with a blender.

2. Season the soup with nutmeg and cayenne, and possibly somewhat salt and pepper.

3. Include emmenthal cheddar and chives and mix a couple of moments until the soup is smooth and prepared to serve. Enhance it with pumpkin seeds.

Nutrition:

Calories: 65

Carbohydrates: 13g

Fat: 2g

Protein: 1g

Lemon-Tarragon Soup

Preparation Time: 10 minutes

Cooking Time: 10 minutes

Servings: 1-2

Cashews and coconut milk replace heavy cream in this healthy version of lemon-tarragon soup, balanced by tart freshly squeezed lemon juice and fragrant tarragon. It's a light, airy soup that you won't want to miss.

Ingredients :

• 1 tablespoon avocado oil

• ½ cup diced onion

• 3 garlic cloves, crushed

• ¼ plus ⅛ teaspoon sea salt

• ¼ plus ⅛ teaspoon freshly ground black pepper

• 1 (13.5-ounce) can full-fat coconut milk

• 1 tablespoon freshly squeezed lemon juice

• ½ cup raw cashews

• 1 celery stalk

• 2 tablespoons chopped fresh tarragon

Directions:

1. In a medium skillet over medium-high warmth, heat the avocado oil. Add the onion, garlic, salt, and pepper, and sauté for 3 to 5 minutes or until the onion is soft.

2. In a high-speed blender, blend together the coconut milk, lemon juice, cashews, celery, and tarragon with the onion mixture until smooth. Adjust seasonings, if necessary.

3. Fill 1 huge or 2 little dishes and enjoy immediately, or transfer to a medium saucepan and warm on low heat for 3 to 5 minutes before serving.

Nutrition:

Calories: 60

Carbohydrates: 13 g

Protein: 0.8 g

Chilled Cucumber And Lime Soup

Preparation Time: 5 minutes

Cooking Time: 20 minutes

Servings: 1-2

Ingredients :

• 1 cucumber, peeled

• ½ zucchini, peeled

• 1 tablespoon freshly squeezed lime juice

• 1 tablespoon fresh cilantro leaves

• 1 garlic clove, crushed

• ¼ teaspoon sea salt

Directions:

1. In a blender, blend together the cucumber, zucchini, lime juice, cilantro, garlic, and salt until well combined. Add more salt, if necessary.

2. Fill 1 huge or 2 little dishes and enjoy immediately, or refrigerate for 15 to 20 minutes to chill before serving.

Nutrition:

Calories: 48

Carbohydrates: 8 g

Fat: 1g

Protein: .5g

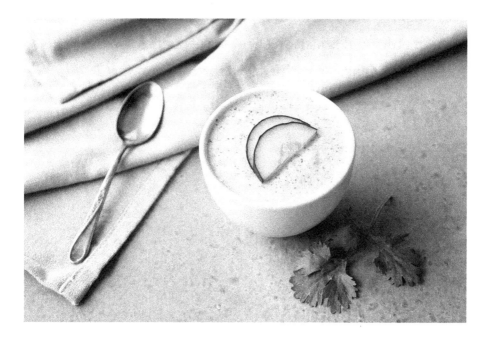

Coconut, Cilantro, And Jalapeño Soup

Preparation Time: 5 minutes

Cooking Time: 5 minutes

Servings: 1-2

This soup is a nutrient dream. Cilantro is a natural anti-inflammatory and is also excellent for detoxification. And one single jalapeño has an entire day's worth of vitamin C!

Ingredients :

- 2 tablespoons avocado oil

- ½ cup diced onions

- 3 garlic cloves, crushed

- ¼ teaspoon sea salt

- 1 (13.5-ounce) can full-fat coconut milk

- 1 tablespoon freshly squeezed lime juice

- ½ to 1 jalapeño

- 2 tablespoons fresh cilantro leaves

Directions:

1. In a medium skillet over medium-high warmth, heat the avocado oil. Include the garlic, onion salt, and pepper, and sauté for 3 to 5 minutes, or until the onions are soft.

2. In a blender, blend together the coconut milk, lime juice, jalapeño, and cilantro with the onion mixture until creamy.

3. Fill 1 huge or 2 little dishes and enjoy.

Nutrition:

Calories: 75

Carbohydrates: 13 g

Fat: 2 g

Protein: 4 g

Spicy Watermelon Gazpacho

Preparation Time: 5 minutes
Cooking Time: 5 minutes
Servings: 1-2

At first taste, this soup may have you wondering if you're lunching on a hot and spicy salsa. It has the heat and seasonings of a traditional tomato-based salsa, but it also has a faint sweetness from the cool watermelon. The soup is really hot with a whole jalapeño, so if you don't like food too hot, just use half a jalapeño.

Ingredients :

• 2 cups cubed watermelon

• ¼ cup diced onion

• ¼ cup packed cilantro leaves

• ½ to 1 jalapeño

• 2 tablespoons freshly squeezed lime juice

Directions:

1. In a blender or food processor, pulse to combine the watermelon, onion, cilantro, jalapeño, and lime juice only long enough to break down the Ingredients, leaving them very finely diced and taking care to not over process.

2. Pour into 1 large or 2 small bowls and enjoy.

Nutrition:

Calories: 35

Carbohydrates: 12

Fat: .4 g

Roasted Carrot and Leek Soup

Preparation Time: 4 minutes
Cooking Time: 30 minutes
Servings: 3-4

The carrot, a root vegetable, is an excellent source of antioxidants (1 cup has 113 percent of your daily value of vitamin A) and fibre (1 cup has 14 percent of your daily value). This bright and colourful soup freezes well to enjoy later when you're short on time.

Ingredients :

• 6 carrots

• 1 cup chopped onion

• 1 fennel bulb, cubed

• 2 garlic cloves, crushed

• 2 tablespoons avocado oil

• 1 teaspoon sea salt

• 1 teaspoon freshly ground black pepper

• 2 cups almond milk, plus more if desired

Directions:

1. Preheat the oven to 400°F. Line a baking sheet with parchment paper.

2. Cut the carrots into thirds, and then cut each third in half. Transfer to a medium bowl.

3. Add the onion, fennel, garlic, and avocado oil, and toss to coat. Season with the salt and pepper, and toss again.

4. Transfer the vegetables to the prepared baking sheet, and roast for 30 minutes.

5. Remove from the oven and allow the vegetables to cool.

6. In a high-speed blender, blend together the almond milk and roasted vegetables until creamy and smooth. Adjust the seasonings, if necessary, and add additional milk if you prefer a thinner consistency.

7. Pour into 2 large or 4 small bowls and enjoy.

Nutrition:

Calories: 55

Carbohydrates: 12g

Fat: 1.5 g

Protein: 1.8 g

Creamy Lentil And Potato Stew

Preparation Time: 10 minutes
Cooking Time: 30 minutes
Servings: 4

This is a hearty stew that is sure to be a favourite. It's a one-pot meal that is the perfect comfort food. With fresh vegetables and herbs along with protein-rich lentils, it's both healthy and filling. Any lentil variety would work, even a mixed, sprouted lentil blend. Another bonus of this recipe: It's freezer-friendly.

Ingredients :

• 2 tablespoons avocado oil

• ½ cup diced onion

• 2 garlic cloves, crushed

• 1 to 1½ teaspoons sea salt

• 1 teaspoon freshly ground black pepper

• 1 cup dry lentils

• 2 carrots, sliced

• 1 cup peeled and cubed potato

- 1 celery stalk, diced

- 2 fresh oregano sprigs, chopped

- 2 fresh tarragon sprigs, chopped

- 5 cups vegetable broth, divided

- 1 (13.5-ounce) can full-fat coconut milk

Directions:

1. In a great soup pot over average-high hotness, heat the avocado oil. Include the garlic, onion, salt, and pepper, and sauté for 3 to 5 minutes, or until the onion is soft.

2. Add the lentils, carrots, potato, celery, oregano, tarragon, and 2½ cups of vegetable broth, and stir.

3. Get to a boil, decrease the heat to medium-low, and cook, stirring frequently and adding additional vegetable broth a half cup at a time to make sure there is enough liquid for the lentils and potatoes to cook, for 20 to 25 minutes, or until the potatoes and lentils are soft.

4. Take away from the heat, and stirring in the coconut milk. Pour into 4 soup bowls and enjoy.

Nutrition:

Calories: 85

Carbohydrates: 20g

Fat: 3g

Protein: 3g

Roasted Garlic And Cauliflower Soup

Preparation Time: 10 minutes

Cooking Time: 35 minutes

Servings: 1-2

Roasted garlic is always a treat, and paired with cauliflower in this wonderful soup, what you get is a deeply satisfy soup with savoury, rustic flavors. Blended, the result is a smooth, thick, and creamy soup, but if you prefer a thinner consistency, just adds a little more vegetable broth to thin it out. Cauliflower is anti-inflammatory, high in antioxidants, and a good source of vitamin C (1 cup has 86 percent of your daily value).

Ingredients :

• 4 cups bite-size cauliflower florets

• 5 garlic cloves

• 1½ tablespoons avocado oil

• ¾ teaspoon sea salt

• ½ teaspoon freshly ground black pepper

• 1 cup almond milk

• 1 cup vegetable broth, plus more if desired

Directions:

1. Preheat the oven to 450°F. Line a baking sheet with parchment paper.

2. In a medium bowl, toss the cauliflower and garlic with the avocado oil to coat. Season with the salt and pepper, and toss again.

3. Transfer to the prepared baking sheet and roast for 30 minutes. Cool before adding to the blender.

4. In a high-speed blender, blend together the cooled vegetables, almond milk, and vegetable broth until creamy and smooth. Adjust the salt and pepper, if necessary, and add additional vegetable broth if you prefer a thinner consistency.

5. Transfer to a medium saucepan, and lightly warm on medium-low heat for 3 to 5 minutes.

6. Ladle into 1 large or 2 small bowls and enjoy.

Nutrition:

Calories: 48

Carbohydrates: 11g

Protein: 1.5g

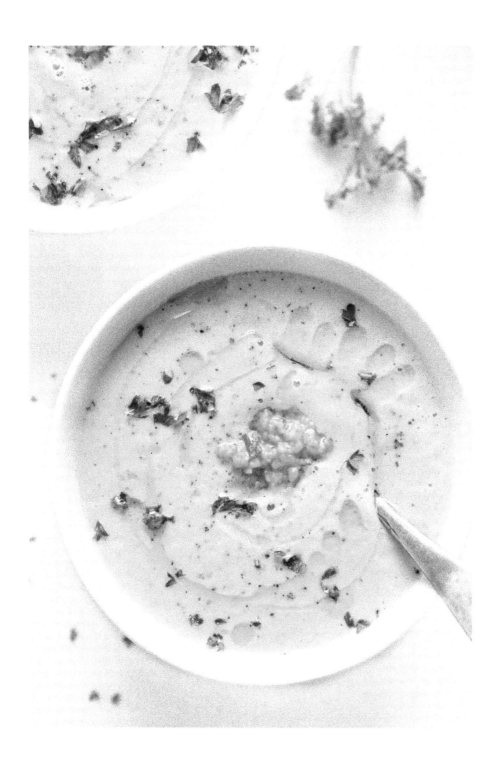

CPSIA information can be obtained
at www.ICGtesting.com
Printed in the USA
BVHW091951180521
607636BV00010B/1256

9 781802 773156